LEARNING
TO LIVE WITH
HYPERTENSION

Revised Edition
A MIPI Publication

The first edition of *Learning to Live with Hypertension* was developed with the help of all these people. We appreciate their efforts, and of all those involved in helping to revise the book for the new edition.

CONSULTANTS

Aram V. Chobanian, M.D., Director, Cardiovascular Institute and Professor of Medicine, Boston University School of Medicine, Boston, Massachusetts

Sue B. Foster, R.N., M.S.N., Director, Nursing Education and Research Program, Beth Israel Hospital, Boston, Massachusetts

John Jainchill, M.D., Internist, The Urban Medical Group, Inc.; Assistant Professor of Socio-Medical Sciences, Boston University School of Medicine, Boston, Massachusetts

Lawrence R. Krakoff, M.D., Professor of Medicine and Chief, Hypertension Division, Mount Sinai School of Medicine of the City University of New York, New York, New York

James O. Taylor, M.D., Medical Director, East Boston Neighborhood Health Center; Associate Clinical Professor of Medicine, Brigham and Women's Hospital and Harvard Medical School, Boston, Massachusetts

PATIENT ADVISERS

Mary Claire Adams, John R. Bailey, Laura Carlson, Calvin Clemons, Azell Davis, and Barbara Droz

SERIES ADVISORY COMMITTEE

Pamela W. Brown, R.N., M.S., Assistant Professor of Nursing, Massachusetts College of Pharmacy and Allied Health Sciences, Boston, Massachusetts

Ralph Hingson, Sc.D., Associate Professor of Socio-Medical Sciences, Boston University Schools of Medicine and Public Health, Boston, Massachusetts

John D. Stoeckle, M.D., Professor of Medicine, Harvard Medical School, and Physician, Massachusetts General Hospital, Boston, Massachusetts

SERIES STAFF

Directors: Judith P. Swazey, Ph.D., President, Acadia Institute, Bar Harbor, Maine; Board of Directors, Medicine In the Public Interest

Louis Lasagna, M.D., Academic Dean, School of Medicine, and Dean, Sackler School of Graduate Biomedical Science, Tufts University, Boston, Massachusetts; President, Board of Directors, Medicine In the Public Interest

Robert J. Levine, M.D., Professor of Medicine, Lecturer in Pharmacology, Yale University School of Medicine, New Haven, Connecticut; Board of Directors, Medicine In the Public Interest

Revised Edition
Writer and Consultant: Judith Fine-Edelstein, M.D.

CONTENTS

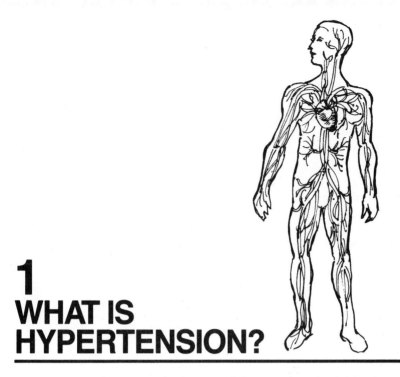

1
WHAT IS HYPERTENSION?

You may have recently discovered that you have high blood pressure (also known as *hypertension*), or you may have had high blood pressure for some period of time. There are likely many questions that you have regarding the meaning of high blood pressure, how high blood pressure is treated and, most importantly, how you can live with it. Even if you are now being treated for high blood pressure, there are probably many questions that you still may have. You may not know what the important questions are that you should ask your doctor, and you may even be anxious about doing so.

In this book, we will explain many important things about high blood pressure. This book is meant to help you better understand what it means to have high blood pressure and how it is treated. It is a guide for you to use in any way that may be helpful to you. All the new information that you learn may stimulate many questions that you can discuss with your doctor, with other health professionals, and with family members. Most importantly, you can become a very active partner in the management of your high blood pressure. We also want to encourage you to play a primary role in other aspects of your health care. To help you do so, we will make you aware of other factors that you can control to help keep yourself in the best health possible.

WHAT IS BLOOD PRESSURE?

In order to understand hypertension, it would be most helpful to learn a little about the important organs in the human body that are involved in controlling blood pressure. After we introduce each organ individually, we can put the big picture together and see how high blood pressure might develop. It is important for you to remember as you are learning this new information that even doctors and scientists who study high blood pressure have questions that still remain unanswered.

The organs in the body that are the most important in blood pressure control are those of the *cardiovascular system* (the heart, and the blood vessels, which carry the blood). We will now explore the way in which these organs function individually and together, and how they relate to blood pressure control.

YOUR HEART

The heart is actually a muscle that is about the size of your fist. It is located in the left side of your chest underneath your rib cage, and is protected by the ribs and tissue coverings. The medical term for the muscular portions of the heart is the *myocardium* ("myo" means "muscle," and "cardium" refers to "heart"). It is a hollow organ that has four separate compartments, each with its own separate function. The heart also has unique parts which are responsible for producing the steady heartbeat that you can feel in your chest and at many other locations in your body. This muscular character of the heart and its ability to beat continuously help the heart to serve as a "pump" which pushes the blood into a series of organs called *blood vessels.*

The heart has four separate sections known as *chambers.* Two of them are known as the *atria* and the other two as the *ventricles.* There is a right and left atrium, and a right and left ventricle. The heart, then, really has two sides: a right side which contains a right atrium and right ventricle, and a left side which contains a left atrium and left ventricle. The structure that separates the atrium on each side from its ventricle is known as a *valve,* similar to valves you might have on machinery in your home. These valves open and close to let blood pass through from an atrium to its ventricle at the appropriate time.

YOUR BLOOD VESSELS

The blood vessels are a long series of an elastic-like system of tubes, whose function is to carry the blood to all of the different organs in your body. For example, blood vessels carry blood to your brain, your kidneys, and to your muscles. This large network of blood vessels is said to be about 70,000 miles long! There are several different kinds of blood vessels which we will discuss, because it is important to understand how the circulatory system really works.

The *arteries* are elastic-like tubes with thick muscular walls that carry the blood from the heart to all of the different organs in your body. The arteries carry the higher-pressure blood coming directly from the heart, therefore their walls are quite thick. They come in all different widths, from the size of a large finger to very narrow arteries about the width of a pencil point. Larger arteries continually branch into smaller ones, until the smallest of all arteries receives your blood. These very small arteries are known as *arterioles*.

A very important artery and the largest in your body is called the *aorta*. It is the artery that receives all of the blood from the heart and sends the blood on its journey to all of the bodily organs. It is located in the left side of your chest.

The *veins* are also tubular structures, but they have much thinner walls than the arteries do because they carry lower-pressure blood back to the heart. They range from very large veins to those that are very small. The smallest of veins are known as *venules*. Just as all of the organs in your body have arteries bringing them blood, each organ has veins which carry the blood from the organs back towards the heart. The veins contain valves that open and close with each heartbeat to prevent blood from flowing in a backwards direction.

The *capillaries* are the tiniest of all of the blood vessels. There are about 10 billion capillaries in your body! They form groups located among all of the organs in the body. They have the thinnest walls of all of the blood vessels we have mentioned so far. Their role is to receive the blood from the smallest arterioles and deliver it to the organs. They also serve to take the blood from the organs and transfer it to the veins, which will eventually bring the blood back towards the heart.

YOUR BLOOD

Blood is a very important substance whose most important function is to deliver oxygen and nutrients to the many organs in your body. It is composed of both fluid components and of red blood cells. These tiny cells have the ability to carry oxygen along and to distribute the oxygen to the organs that need it. Blood also carries other substances, such as nutrients from the foods that we eat, chemicals that the body makes, and even medications which are carried throughout the blood stream to act on different bodily organs. Blood also carries carbon dioxide, which is formed in the bodily organs, and delivers it to the lungs. The total amount of blood in your body varies somewhat with body size, but there are about 8-12 pints that circulate continually throughout your body.

THE CIRCULATORY SYSTEM: PUTTING IT ALL TOGETHER

All of the components we have discussed are responsible for circulating the blood throughout your body. Let's examine them, and follow your blood as it flows through the entire circulatory system.

The heart's thick wall functions as a muscular machine to pump the blood into the blood vessels. As the thick muscular wall contracts, the blood is forced out of the heart and into the blood vessels. The heart beats an average of 70 times a minute, but this varies from person to person. Over a full day of 24 hours, this comes to about 100,000 beats per day! The heart pumps approximately 2-3 ounces of blood with each beat, and a total of 2,000 gallons of blood each day.

Let's look at the blood in the left ventricle of your heart. The journey begins here. The thick heart-muscle wall contracts, forcing the blood out of the left ventricle and into the largest artery in your body, the aorta. The blood is then continually pumped, with each heartbeat, through the series of arteries, to all of the organs. The blood travels through smaller and smaller arterioles to reach the capillary bed which, through its tiny thin walls, delivers the oxygen carried by the red blood cells and other nutrients in the blood to the organs. It is here that the blood picks up carbon dioxide formed in the organs.

After these nutrients and oxygen are deposited, the blood begins its journey back towards the heart, first through the capillary bed and then through larger and larger veins until the blood reaches the right side of the heart. The blood first enters the right atrium then passes through one of the valves to the right ventricle. From here, it is pumped through the lungs. The function of the lungs is to give oxygen back to the blood and to clear the carbon dioxide that the blood has been carrying from the various bodily organs. From the lungs, the blood is pumped into the left side of the heart into the left atrium. It is then pumped into the left ventricle where we started and pumped back into the blood vessels to repeat the journey.

Although we followed the blood from the left ventricle through its course, the two sides of the heart actually pump at the same time. The two atria contract at the same time, forcing blood into the two ventricles. When the atria relax, the blood is pumped from both sides of the heart by the two ventricles—from the right ventricle through the heart to obtain oxygen and deposit carbon dioxide in the lungs, and from the left ventricle to the arterial system to reach all of the bodily organs.

Now that you understand how the circulatory system functions, we can begin to explore what blood pressure is and why it might be elevated.

YOUR BLOOD PRESSURE

As the heart pumps the blood through the blood vessels, the blood comes in contact with the walls of these vessels. The force of the blood against the artery walls is known as *blood pressure*. When the heart contracts and is actively pumping blood through the vessels, the force on the walls of the arteries increases. When the heart is relaxed (in between heartbeats) the pressure on the walls of these vessels is decreased. So, you see, even within one heartbeat cycle the blood pressure varies, depending upon whether the heart is contracting or not. Your blood pressure, then, is really a measure of the force that your blood places against the walls of your arteries.

When the heart is contracting, this phase of the cycle is known as *systole*. During systole, the heart pumps blood out of the ventricles. After this contraction, the ventricles fill with blood from the atria. This phase of the heart's cycle is known as *diastole*. The reason why these two phases are important is that the medical terms for the two numbers reported in your blood pressure measurement are known as *systolic* and *diastolic,* referring to these two phases in the cardiac cycle. We will be discussing measuring your blood pressure in more detail in the next section.

Your blood pressure can vary depending on the time of the day, the activities that you are involved in, or even how you are feeling. For example, in times of great stress or when you are anxious, your blood pressure can go up. Blood pressure can also rise during periods of exercise, and fall when you are at rest. Exercise, however, is an important part of a healthy life for many people, and we will discuss the benefits of exercise in other sections of this book.

HOW DOES YOUR BODY CONTROL YOUR BLOOD PRESSURE?

Your blood pressure is controlled by very complex mechanisms in your body that involve many different organs. These include your *nervous system* (your brain and the nerves throughout the body), your kidneys, and your *hormones* (special bodily chemicals released into the blood circulation that have different effects on the body). As you can imagine, your body has to control your blood pressure quickly over the short term, such as in times of stress or exercise, and over the long term throughout your lifetime. Your blood pressure ensures that blood flows to all the organs in your body, supplying them with the oxygen and nutrients that they need.

There is a specific range of blood pressure that your system strives to maintain. Your nervous system and hormones are mostly involved in short-term blood pressure control. Your kidneys, by controlling the fluid and *salt* (sodium) in your body, are mostly involved in long-term control over blood pressure.

In order to maintain your blood pressure over the short term, special sensors are located along arteries in your neck. These sensors send information about your blood pressure through special nerves to specific parts of the brain. The brain sends hormones into the circulation. These hormones can act on different aspects of your circulatory system—for example, on your arteries, to control your blood pressure. If your sensors indicate that your blood pressure is too low, the hormones released will act on your arteries and cause them to *constrict* (or tighten). This results in increased resistance to blood flowing through the arteries, which increases your blood pressure. Similarly, hormones can act upon blood vessels to *dilate* them (make the width greater) if your blood pressure becomes high. As your blood vessels widen, your blood pressure goes down. This system can act within seconds to keep your blood pressure within a steady range.

Your kidneys also play a very important role in long-term blood pressure control. The body has two kidneys. There is one on each side, located deep within your body behind the digestive organs toward your back. Although the function of the kidneys is very complex, with regard to blood pressure control they mainly serve to regulate the amount of fluid and salt in your body. When blood pressure is too high, the kidneys can help the body get rid of fluid and salt, which can then result in a lower blood pressure. On the other hand, when the pressure is low, the body can hold on to salt and fluid, thereby raising the blood pressure. The retention of water and salt is controlled by special bodily chemicals that act on the kidneys.

These mechanisms of blood pressure control work automatically. There are also other factors that help control blood pressure. These include your heart's ability to pump your blood effectively, plus the volume of blood in your body. Blood pressure is also kept in a healthy range by the action of your muscles working on your veins to push the blood back towards the heart so that it circulates more rapidly.

Now that we have described the bodily systems involved in the production and the control of your blood pressure, we can explore the concept of *hypertension* (high blood pressure). In chapters to come, we will be examining the causes of hypertension, risk factors, and the treatment strategies doctors use to control high blood pressure. Most importantly, we will be focusing on how to help you live with your hypertension and stay as healthy as you can be.

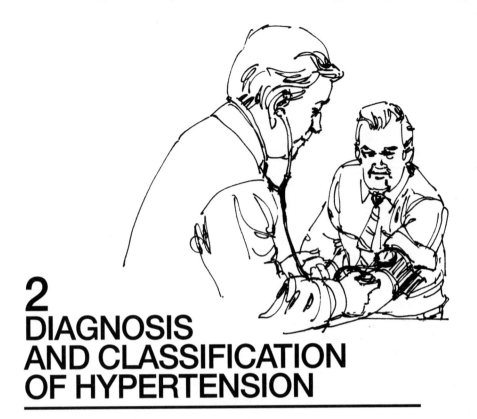

2
DIAGNOSIS
AND CLASSIFICATION
OF HYPERTENSION

How does your doctor determine that your blood pressure is high? Where do the numbers come from and just what do they mean? Does your doctor need other medical information in addition to your blood pressure to decide upon appropriate treatment?

In this chapter we will describe how your doctor will take your blood pressure and what the numbers really mean. We will define hypertension and classify high blood pressure into different categories.

Blood pressure is the force your blood applies against your artery walls. Hypertension (high blood pressure) implies that this pressure is increased. We have seen that the body has a very organized system whereby blood pressure is controlled. It is normal, however, for blood pressure to fluctuate during the day. At different times, we all may have "high blood pressure" for short periods. The body's control system is usually able to regulate these ups and downs in the blood pressure.

When your doctor makes a diagnosis of hypertension, it means that the arterial blood pressure is higher than the upper accepted range for normal blood pressure. Hypertension is diagnosed by measuring a series of several blood pressure readings which are taken several days or weeks apart. It is important for your doctor to obtain a range of readings to diagnose hypertension accurately. Your doctor must be sure that your blood pressure was not just mildly elevated as part of the normal ups and downs of pressure during the day. It is quite common for your blood pressure to be higher in the doctor's office because it is often very hard to relax there, so your doctor will measure a pattern of blood pressure and then decide upon the appropriate treatment. Sometimes, however, your doctor may rely on a single blood pressure reading. If this reading is extremely high, it may need to be addressed without waiting to take additional blood pressure readings.

MEASURING YOUR BLOOD PRESSURE

Your doctor or other health professional has probably taken your blood pressure many times on past examinations. Most doctors use the same method of blood pressure determination. The most common measurement device used today is called a *sphygmomanometer* (sfig-moe-muh-nom-eh-ter). The name means "measuring the pulse" and the device is also known as the "blood pressure cuff."

It has several important parts you should know about. There is a cloth or rubber cuff which is wrapped around your arm. It is attached to a hose with a small rubber air bulb that is used to pump air into the cuff. A *manometer* (a glass tube similar to a thermometer) which has numbers that indicate the blood pressure reading is also attached to the system. Some systems may have variations in the meter used to register the blood pressure reading. The other important piece of equipment used to take your blood pressure is a *stethoscope*, which is used to hear your pulse so your blood pressure can be recorded.

The cuff is placed around your bare upper arm just above the bend in your elbow. One end of the stethoscope is placed in your doctor's or nurse's ears, while the other end is placed just over the crease in your arm beneath the cuff. There is an artery located here with blood circulating through that will provide the sounds necessary to determine your blood pressure. The bulb is squeezed slowly as the cuff becomes inflated with air. Air is continually pumped into the cuff pressing on the artery in your arm until it temporarily stops the blood from flowing into this artery. The manometer continually measures the elevated pressure as the air is pumped into the cuff.

Initially, enough air is pumped into the cuff to bring the manometer reading way above your real blood pressure. No sounds are heard through the stethoscope that is placed on your artery because there is no blood flowing through at this time. Your doctor or nurse then very slowly begins to let the air out of the cuff by opening the valve on the hand-held pump. As this air is let out, the reading on the manometer begins to fall. It is at this time that the first of two blood pressure sounds is heard. The blood that was initially prevented from flowing through the artery by the tight cuff now begins to flow towards your forearm. Your doctor or nurse listens carefully for the beating of your pulse as they let air out of the cuff. They will record the number displayed on the manometer at the time they hear this first sound. This sound is your *systolic* blood pressure. It occurs at the time the pressure in the cuff is just lower than the pressure in your artery. As more air is let out of the cuff, the manometer reading continues to fall. Your doctor or nurse will continue to hear your pulse as they continue to let the air out of the cuff. When they no longer can hear any pulse, they will record the reading on the manometer and record this as your *diastolic* pressure. Like old-fashioned thermometers, manometers contain mercury inside a glass column. The mercury moves up and down the column. There are millimeter measures alongside the column of mercury. Thus, if your systolic blood pressure is 140, this means that it would take a pressure of 140 to raise a column of mercury to 140 mm.

What does systolic and diastolic blood pressure really mean? Why are two numbers needed to describe your blood pressure?

When we described the function of your heart, we divided the heart's pumping cycle into two phases. The first we called *systolic*, the phase when the heart contracted and pumped its blood out from its ventricles. The second phase is the *diastolic* phase, and represents the heart's relaxation phase, after contraction, when it refills with blood.

The *systolic* blood pressure (the first sound heard when air is let out of the cuff) represents the maximum pressure exerted by blood on your arteries when the heart is contracting. The *diastolic* pressure (recorded when the pulse is no longer heard as air is being let out of the cuff) represents the pressure along the walls of the arteries when the heart is at rest and is refilling with blood.

Your blood pressure, then, is described and recorded as two numbers. The accepted method is to write the blood pressure as the systolic pressure/diastolic pressure; for example, if your blood pressure is 140/90, it is said to be "one-forty over ninety." These are just the technical and scientific definitions of blood pressure. The most important things that you should remember are what your blood pressure readings are, how they relate to your health, and how you can maintain the best health possible.

CLASSIFICATION OF HIGH BLOOD PRESSURE

Although there is still no clear agreement on which specific numbers mean that you have high blood pressure, it is probably useful to have some normal blood pressure readings for comparison. For many years, the common "normal" blood pressure reading for adults was said to be 120/80. There is, however, a range of blood pressure that is considered to be within normal range. For example, many people have blood pressure readings that are lower than 120/80; they may be very healthy but simply have a lower blood pressure.

Most doctors agree that a systolic blood pressure of less than 140 would fall into a normal range; a normal diastolic pressure would be one that is less than or equal to 90. Blood pressure recordings of 140/90 suggest the presence of mild hypertension. Sometimes these readings are referred to as *borderline*, or stage 1 hypertension.

Some doctors believe that blood pressure measurements from 140/90 to 165/100 represent mild-to-moderate, or stage 2 or stage 3 hypertension. Blood pressure readings above these values would be classified as moderate-to-severe, or stage 4 hypertension.

There are two other terms used to describe blood pressure that you should know. The first is a form of severe hypertension that comes on rapidly, bringing blood pressure up to very high levels. It is often known as *malignant hypertension*. (Although you may have heard the word "malignant" in reference to cancer, the word "malignant" here refers solely to the dangerously high level of the blood pressure.) Malignant hypertension is a medical emergency, because the extremely high level of blood pressure can cause severe damage to other bodily organs, including the brain, the kidneys, and the eyes. Death can occur if this condition is not treated.

The second term used to describe blood pressure is *labile hypertension*. This is not really another kind of blood pressure, but the term "labile" refers to the fact that blood pressure can go up and down between levels that are considered "normal" and levels that are considered "high." The high readings tend to occur during times of stress. If your doctor finds that your blood pressure is labile, he or she may want to monitor any high readings closely. Some doctors will consider those with labile hypertension as having *borderline hypertension*. About 10-25% of those who have labile blood pressure will eventually develop definite hypertension.

Here are a few very important points to know:

• There is no clear dividing line between "normal" blood pressure and "high" blood pressure. Researchers have found, however, that the blood pressure levels that are too "high" are those that begin to cause complications. We will be discussing the complications of hypertension in chapters to come.

• Your doctor will take many things into consideration when making a diagnosis of high blood pressure. These include age, race, whether you are male or female, and your general medical condition.

• Doctors previously thought that the diastolic blood pressure (the lower number) was the most important indicator of hypertension and paid most of their attention to this number. Today, we have learned that the systolic blood pressure (the higher number) is equally important in determining how blood pressure should be treated.

• The most important thing to realize is that few people with hypertension actually have daily symptoms of high blood pressure. Unlike other diseases or conditions, you may never feel that anything is wrong. For example, you know when you have a headache because you feel an uncomfortable, painful sensation in your head. You may feel symptoms of a stomach ulcer by noting irritation in your stomach. For these conditions, you may seek medical help and might be treated with medication. With high blood pressure, you may not notice any particular daily symptoms of pain or discomfort for a long period of time or until the damage to bodily organs from hypertension occurs. A few people may have symptoms such as headache, dizziness, or even nosebleeds. Hypertension, however, is often discovered during a routine medical evaluation. The absence of any symptoms should not surprise you.

In addition to blood pressure recordings, your doctor may perform a series of tests as part of the diagnostic evaluation of persons with hypertension. These will help determine your general medical health, as well as determine any other related medical conditions or complications from the hypertension.

THE OFFICE VISIT

After your doctor discovers that you have high blood pressure, he or she will perform a thorough physical examination and take a careful medical history from you.

YOUR MEDICAL HISTORY

Your doctor or nurse will obtain a thorough medical history from you to get a picture of how your health has been over your lifetime. This medical history will provide your doctor with very useful information. You will be asked whether anyone has ever discovered that your blood pressure has been high in the past, or whether you have ever been treated for high blood pressure. You will be asked whether you have had any symptoms which may suggest complications of high blood pressure such as severe headaches, nosebleeds, or dizziness. You will be asked about other medical problems such as heart disease, kidney disease, lung disease, or diabetes. You will be asked whether you have ever had a stroke, or blood vessel problems in other parts of your body. You will be asked about any medications you may be taking. It is important to tell your doctor about all medications that you may be using, including over-the-counter cold remedies, diet aids, or birth control pills.

You will be asked about the health of your family members, including your parents and siblings. Your doctor will specifically be interested in any family history of high blood pressure, heart disease, kidney disease, stroke, or similar diseases. Your doctor will take a detailed family history from you, as high blood pressure can be hereditary in some cases. You will also be asked questions about your lifestyle. These will include questions about your dietary habits, your level of physical activity, your employment history, and your relationships with family and friends. In general, your doctor will have an impression of how things in your life are going.

YOUR PHYSICAL EXAMINATION

The purpose of the physical examination is for your doctor to know your state of health. Your doctor will be looking for any indication that there have been complications from your hypertension. Your weight will be taken; your blood pressure will be measured.

One way your doctor can determine if there has been any damage to your bodily organs from hypertension is to look into your eyes. By using an *ophthalmoscope* (an instrument that permits your doctor to look at the small blood vessels in the retina, in the back portion of your eye), your doctor can detect changes that may have been the result of high blood pressure. These are the only blood vessels that your doctor can see from the outside. These small arteries and veins are important because in many ways they are similar to other blood vessels in your body. If early changes from high blood pressure are detected here, it may indicate that other blood vessels are also affected.

Your doctor will palpate your heart by placing his or her hands on your chest. The stethoscope will be used to listen to your heart. The sounds of the heart valves and flowing blood will help determine the pumping function of your heart. The stethoscope will also be used to listen to your lungs, to assure that there is not any fluid present. These findings may indicate that your heart may have been affected by high blood pressure.

Your doctor will feel your pulse in many different areas of your body. These include the pulses in your feet and legs, in your groin, in your abdominal cavity, and in your neck. The stethoscope will also be used to listen to some of these blood vessels for signs of narrowing, which may result in a decrease in blood flow. Your abdomen will be examined for abnormal signs in your kidneys or liver. Your doctor will look for indications of swelling or other changes in your skin. Other parts of the physical exam may be performed if your doctor feels they are necessary.

LABORATORY TESTING

Your doctor may want to obtain some general blood tests at the time of your physical examination. These include tests of your red and white blood cells, analysis of your kidney and liver function, an evaluation of your blood *glucose* (sugar) level, and tests to determine your cholesterol and other blood *lipids* (blood fats). If your doctor suspects that your hypertension may be due to a specific disorder of your kidneys, or of your *adrenal glands* (small glands positioned above the kidneys), further laboratory testing may be performed.

Your doctor will also obtain a urine sample and perform a urinalysis looking for glucose or proteins in the urine. This will provide information on the function of your kidneys. Other specific tests can be performed on your urine if your doctor feels they are necessary.

THE ELECTROCARDIOGRAM

The *electrocardiogram,* also known as the *EKG* or the *ECG,* is commonly performed during medical office visits. It is a simple means of determining many things about the function of the heart and providing information about the *rhythm* (beat) of the heart. Your doctor or your nurse will perform the EKG by placing small round discs (known as the EKG leads) on your arms, legs, and across your chest above the position of your heart. These are connected by thin wires to the main machine, which then transmits the signal to a pen, which traces the electrical activity of the heart onto a strip of moving paper. Each heartbeat (which represents the heart's muscular contraction) appears on the paper strip as a particular pattern in a wave that your doctor can then analyze.

The EKG can provide your doctor with information about the size of some of the chambers of the heart. It can indicate whether there has been any damage to the heart. Your doctor can also monitor the rhythm of your heart during the EKG to assure that the heartbeat is regular and beating at a normal rate.

Your doctor may also decide to obtain other tests during your physical examination. These may include a chest x-ray or an echocardiogram.

A *chest x-ray* will provide your doctor with an actual x-ray picture of your chest and the organs it contains, namely, the heart and the lungs. The x-ray shows a rough estimate of the size and shape of the heart. The heart can be enlarged as a result of high blood pressure, and your doctor would want this information. The x-ray also shows the lungs clearly and will let your doctor know if fluid (which may be the result of poor heart function) has collected in the lungs. This is known as *congestive heart failure* and will be described in future chapters.

An *echocardiogram* is a procedure used to evaluate the structure and the function of the heart. This test uses high frequency sound waves (known as *ultrasound*) to show an actual image of the heart. A small instrument is placed on your chest which bounces sound waves off the different parts of your heart. As it scans your heart, the image is formed on a screen. This test can provide information about the size of your heart, its pumping function, and the condition of its valves (which we have previously described as the parts of the heart that let the blood flow from one chamber to another).

Now that you are familiar with how your doctor will diagnose hypertension and what the physical examination and laboratory evaluation might be like, we can explore hypertension itself in more detail. In the next chapter, we will focus on some of the risk factors associated with hypertension.

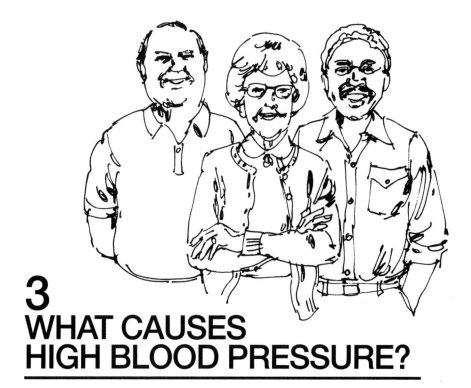

3
WHAT CAUSES HIGH BLOOD PRESSURE?

High blood pressure is the most common long-term medical condition in the United States. In fact, many millions of Americans have high blood pressure. In 90-95% of those who have high blood pressure, the cause is unknown. This form of high blood pressure is often called *primary* or *essential* hypertension because the mechanism that causes the increase in blood pressure is unknown. When there is a known cause for the high blood pressure, it is often called *secondary* hypertension because it is thought to be secondary to particular medical disorders.

ESSENTIAL HYPERTENSION

Essential hypertension is the form of high blood pressure that is found in more than 90% of people who have high blood pressure. Even though there is no clear cause, there are certain common characteristics found in many patients who have this form of high blood pressure. Certain risk factors can increase the chance of developing hypertension. It is important to remember that these risk factors do not clearly <u>cause</u> hypertension but are common in many individuals <u>with</u> hypertension. They are very important to identify because some of them can be modified and may result in lowering the blood pressure.

Age

Although people of any age can develop high blood pressure, it is found more commonly in older individuals. While high blood pressure is often diagnosed when people are between the ages of 35-50, in many individuals a pattern of consistently increased blood pressure is not noted until they are much older. The younger a person is when they have high blood pressure diagnosed, the shorter their life can be expected to be if it is left untreated. For these reasons it is extremely important to treat high blood pressure.

Sex

For people under the age of 50, high blood pressure is more common in men, although it occurs about equally in both sexes by the age of 55. In general, females at all ages tend to do better and have fewer deaths from the complications of hypertension than men.

Race

In the United States, blacks have twice the likelihood of developing high blood pressure than do whites. Blacks also tend to develop high blood pressure at a younger age, have higher levels of blood pressure, and are four times as likely to develop complications from hypertension as compared to whites.

Heredity

Heredity refers to the fact that some diseases can run in families. Doctors find that many people with hypertension seem to have other family members who also have high blood pressure. Because it is such a common medical disorder, however, it is not clear how important a family history of high blood pressure really is in most cases. Having a family history of hypertension probably interacts with other factors to result in high blood pressure.

Weight

There is a definite relationship between being overweight and having high blood pressure. Gaining weight is often associated with an increase in blood pressure in people who previously had normal blood pressure, and approximately 40% of people who are overweight have high blood pressure. The good news is that when overweight people lose weight, there is often a decrease in their blood pressure. If they are also being treated with medication, losing weight also makes it easier to control blood pressure. Remember, though, that you can have high blood pressure even if you are not overweight.

Environment

We all know the feeling of being stressed. Although there is no clear proof that a stressful environment can cause high blood pressure, some researchers feel there is a connection between our stress levels and blood pressure levels. Other factors that have been looked into and may be related to developing high blood pressure include family size and the home environment, job occupation, and general lifestyle. It is often hard to separate the environmental factors from those related to a family history of hypertension because families often share the same lifestyle.

Dietary Habits

One important factor that seems to relate to the development of high blood pressure in some individuals is the amount of their salt intake. In some people with hypertension, eating salty foods can increase their blood pressure and make it more difficult to control. Others may be able to eat foods with salt without developing problems. Your doctor will let you know the importance of a strict diet in your case.

These risk factors do not necessarily <u>cause</u> hypertension, but many of them may interact together in some individuals. In others who have high blood pressure, there may not be any clear risk factors evident. Some risk factors can be modified, while others, such as age, race and sex, cannot be controlled. We will discuss different ways to modify some of these factors in future chapters.

SECONDARY HYPERTENSION

This form of high blood pressure is "secondary" to some other disease process. It is much less common than essential hypertension and occurs in less than 10% of people who have high blood pressure. It is very important to search for potential causes of high blood pressure because with treatment of the underlying cause, in some cases the hypertension can be cured. Some of the more common disorders that may be responsible for secondary hypertension include kidney and endocrine disease.

Hypertension Due to Kidney Disease

The kidneys are a very important set of organs that help regulate body fluids, as well as the amount of sodium and potassium in the blood stream. Changes in blood and fluid volume that can occur if the kidneys are not functioning properly can affect blood pressure. In addition, the arteries that supply blood to the kidneys are important parts of the blood pressure regulation system. In certain conditions, the arteries may become very narrow, which can also result in high blood pressure. There are tests that can help diagnose these conditions, as well as some specific treatments that physicians will use in appropriate patients.

Hypertension Due to Endocrine Disease

The endocrine system is made up of your body's hormones and of certain glands such as the *thyroid gland* and the *adrenal glands* (the latter located above the kidneys). These hormones are chemical substances released from the glands into the blood stream. Each hormone has a specific function, and when some hormones are released in large amounts due to specific medical disorders, hypertension can result. In one uncommon disorder, for example, a small abnormal growth in the adrenal glands can release substances that cause the blood pressure to be very high. There are tests to help diagnose these conditions. Treatments that are directed at the primary medical condition can then help to lower the high blood pressure caused by that condition.

There are other diseases that can cause high blood pressure. If your doctor suspects that one of them may be the cause of your high blood pressure, appropriate diagnostic tests will be done. In most cases of high blood pressure, however, there is no clear underlying cause to be found.

Why is it so important to treat high blood pressure? The next chapter will focus on the short- and long-term effects of untreated high blood pressure on your body.

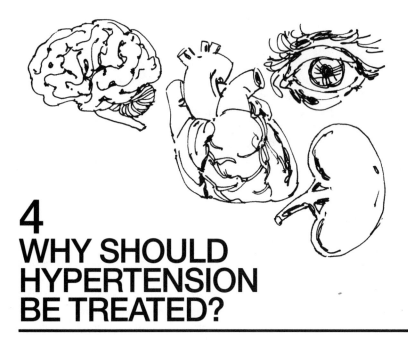

4
WHY SHOULD HYPERTENSION BE TREATED?

One of the most common questions that patients often ask is, "Why should my high blood pressure be treated if I feel OK?" Unfortunately, high blood pressure can exist for many years and you may not feel any symptoms, but during this time the high blood pressure can cause many complications to body systems. The main reason for treating high blood pressure is to prevent the consequences that can develop after years of untreated hypertension.

An important system that is affected by high blood pressure is the *cardiovascular system.* It is composed of the heart and blood vessels that supply blood to the different organs in the body. Other important organs such as the brain, the kidneys, and the eyes can also be damaged by high blood pressure. It is also known that people with hypertension have a shorter life expectancy than those with "normal" blood pressure. For these people, the most common cause of death is heart disease.

In this chapter we will explore the effects of untreated hypertension, stressing the importance of treating it. Our purpose is not to frighten you, but to help you understand how important it is to treat your high blood pressure and control the other risk factors that can be modified. We will also describe other cardiovascular diseases related to high blood pressure. Most importantly, we will focus on the role you can play to help maintain the best health possible.

CARDIOVASCULAR DISEASE

A very important potential consequence of untreated high blood pressure is its effect on the cardiovascular system. As a matter of fact, high blood pressure is thought to be the most important risk factor associated with cardiovascular diseases.

What diseases affect the cardiovascular system and how is high blood pressure involved? In the next section we will describe the effects of hypertension on the cardiovascular system. In future sections we will relate other risk factors to these diseases and focus on how you can play an important role in controlling some of the factors that are related to these diseases.

BLOOD VESSELS AND HYPERTENSION

Over many years, high blood pressure can affect the blood vessels throughout your body. Normally, these vessels have a smooth lining and are relatively elastic, with a muscular wall that allows the blood to move through freely. With normal aging, there is a slow thickening of the walls in these blood vessels. Very slowly over time, with the normal process of aging, fatty materials (such as cholesterol) can build up along the wall of the vessels causing them to be somewhat more rigid.

When blood pressure is high, there is an increased force (or pressure) along all the blood vessels in the body. This can cause injury to the vessels over long periods of time. Fatty materials will clump along the blood vessel's wall. Other blood components can also clump together with the fatty materials creating areas often referred to as *plaques*. Over time, if they continue to build up along the blood vessel wall, the inside of the blood vessel (known as the *lumen*) can become very narrow as well as very stiff, making it more difficult for blood to flow through. This process of plaque buildup along the vessel wall is known as *atherosclerosis*.

Although there are some similar changes in blood vessels that occur naturally with aging, high blood pressure can result in more severe and early disease in these vessels. A continuing cycle can develop where the arteries become increasingly more narrow. Blood pressure becomes more elevated, and the blood flow through the vessels is made more difficult. More and more fatty materials are deposited on the blood vessel wall. As the process continues and becomes more severe, the lumen of the blood vessel can eventually become completely blocked. If this occurs, the result can be that the blood flowing through these arteries can no longer reach the organs it was meant to supply, resulting in organ damage. In the heart, it can result in a heart attack; in the brain, it can result in a stroke.

20

Atherosclerosis mainly affects the arteries, although there can also be changes in the veins. Both the large and small arteries can be affected. The aorta, for example, which is the largest artery in the body and is located in your chest and abdominal cavity, can be affected by this process. Weakness in the walls of the aorta can develop, leading to enlargement of this artery. In some cases, surgery is necessary to repair it.

When the process affects the arteries in the legs, it is more difficult for blood to flow through, which can result in poor blood supply to the muscles and other structures in the legs. This form of vascular disease can result in pain in the calves during exercise or even at rest. In some cases, surgery may be necessary to help restore blood flow.

Atherosclerosis also commonly affects those blood vessels (known as the *coronary arteries*) that bring blood to the heart. When these vessels are affected, blood flow to the heart muscle is reduced, which may result in a heart attack. If your doctor discovers that you have atherosclerosis of the blood vessels, he or she may want to perform specific tests to diagnose the degree and location of these changes.

Remember, by treating high blood pressure, you are playing an important role in helping prevent atherosclerosis. There are other important risk factors that are associated with atherosclerosis, such as cigarette smoking and high cholesterol; we will focus on these in future sections of this book.

THE HEART AND HIGH BLOOD PRESSURE

Hypertension can affect the heart in a number of different ways. The most common cause of death in people with hypertension is heart disease. When the process of atherosclerosis affects the blood vessels that supply blood to the heart (the *coronary arteries*), symptoms result because the blood has difficulty flowing through these blood vessels to reach the heart. The term for this form of atherosclerosis (plaque buildup in these vessels) is known as *coronary artery disease.*

CORONARY ARTERY DISEASE

Coronary artery disease is the leading cause of death in men and women over age 45. Since hypertension is a leading risk factor associated with coronary artery disease, you can see how important it is to control high blood pressure.

Coronary artery disease can be associated with a number of different symptoms. Some people may have what is known as *angina pectoris* (pain in the chest). This symptom of chest pain may also occur with pain in the jaw or the left arm (pain is transmitted from the heart), shortness of breath, or sweating. It signals that the heart is temporarily not getting enough blood and oxygen because of blocking of the coronary arteries due to atherosclerosis.

If a decrease in blood flow to the heart continues for a long time, a *myocardial infarction* (heart attack) can occur. Because of a serious lack of blood flow to the heart muscle, the heart is deprived of its needed oxygen and nutrients. This deprivation causes the heart muscle cells to die. A heart attack results in permanent damage to the specific area of the heart that was supplied by the blocked coronary artery.

Symptoms of chest pain should be taken very seriously and always should be evaluated by your doctor. There are specific tests of chemical substances in your blood and other tests of your heart function that will help your doctor determine if you have suffered heart damage. There are also many medications available that can help to increase the supply of blood to the heart in patients who have narrowing of the coronary arteries due to atherosclerosis.

Your doctor may also determine that a procedure to open up the clogged blood vessels (known as *angioplasty*) or a procedure to bypass the narrowed areas (known as *coronary bypass*) may be necessary.

To help prevent any damage to the heart before it occurs, it is most important to take control of your health and to modify any risk factors that may be associated with coronary artery disease.

CONGESTIVE HEART FAILURE

High blood pressure can also affect the heart muscle in other ways. The heart pumps blood into the arteries, which then deliver the blood to the many organs in the body. When the pressure in the blood vessels is elevated, the heart has to do a great deal of extra work in order to pump the blood into these arteries. Over a long period of time, the heart muscle enlarges in order to perform this work. Unlike the muscles in other parts of your body which may enlarge and become stronger, the enlarged heart muscle sooner or later loses its strength and can no longer effectively pump blood into the arteries through the body. The heart is then said to fail. The flow of blood to the different organs in the body slows down and may eventually be insufficient to maintain the organs' good health. When the heart cannot continue to pump the body's fluids, they can eventually back up into the lungs and the other organs. This condition is known as *congestive heart failure.*

In this condition, the body's fluids are not effectively pumped by the heart and can back up and escape from their place inside the blood vessels. When fluids move into the tissues, swelling (known as *edema*) in the legs can occur. When the lungs become congested with fluid, difficulty in breathing may result. The liver and the kidneys can also be damaged in this condition.

Your doctor can diagnose congestive heart failure by performing a detailed physical examination. There are other diagnostic tests to help evaluate the function of your heart. There are also specific medications which can help reduce the hard work of the heart and can help rid the body of the extra fluid that the heart can no longer handle.

Most deaths due to hypertension occur from myocardial infarction (heart attacks) or from congestive heart failure. You can see how important it is to control high blood pressure early, before severe atherosclerosis of the coronary arteries is present and before heart failure occurs.

STROKE AND HIGH BLOOD PRESSURE

Stroke is the third-leading cause of death in the United States. Even if you survive a stroke, it can be devastating. High blood pressure is the leading risk factor associated with stroke. As a matter of fact, many studies have found that the risk of having a stroke is directly related to how high your blood pressure is.

What is a stroke, and what causes a stroke? Are there any warning signs, and can you help prevent strokes?

There are a number of different types of strokes, but all of them result in damage to various parts of the brain. We can broadly subdivide strokes into those that result from lack of oxygen and blood flow to the brain, and those that result from bleeding into the brain. Although they may result from different causes, they have many of the same risk factors associated with them. First, we will describe the types of strokes and warning symptoms that result from a decreased blood flow to the brain, then we will discuss the other type of stroke that results from bleeding into the brain tissue.

We previously described the process of atherosclerosis that affects blood vessels. Atherosclerosis can result in narrowing and even *occlusion* (complete blocking) of the blood vessels, in turn resulting in decreased blood flow to the organs. The arteries that supply the brain with blood can also be affected by atherosclerosis. The two large arteries in the neck that extend up into the brain are known as the *carotid arteries*. They can become progressively narrowed by fatty deposits and clotted substances in the blood (called *thrombi*) that deposit along the artery walls. Small clots known as *emboli* can break off and travel through other arteries up into the brain. If they become lodged in the arteries of the brain they can result in a stroke, because the blood flow to the brain is either reduced or absent in these areas. This is known as *ischemia*. As the carotid arteries narrow, blood flow to the brain is reduced; this may also result in a stroke.

Besides the carotid arteries, other vessels supply blood to the brain and can be involved in this process. In addition, small blood clots can form in the heart under certain conditions and can also travel through brain arteries obstructing blood flow. If the blood flow is restored quickly, or if the emboli only temporarily clog the artery, warning symptoms may occur. These are known as *TIAs,* which stands for *transient ischemic attacks.* Symptoms are *transient* (brief), get better, and are not permanent. They are very important, however, as a warning that a stroke may occur.

What kind of symptoms would you have in a TIA? Although they may vary, there are some common symptoms. These include weakness or paralysis of the face, arm or leg; numbness or tingling in the face, arm or leg; slurred speech or language problems, loss of vision in one eye, double vision, or dizziness/vertigo. When these events do not get better, the result is a stroke. In a stroke, the blood flow was not restored to the brain and permanent damage has already occurred. To help prevent a stroke, it is very important to seek medical attention immediately if any of these symptoms occur.

Another type of stroke known as a *cerebral hemorrhage* results from bleeding into the brain. The most common form of hemorrhage results from hypertension. The stroke symptoms that we described above can also occur in this condition. In addition, loss of consciousness and coma may occur with hemorrhage into the brain. TIAs usually do not occur prior to this form of stroke, so there are no warning signs in most cases.

If your doctor determines that you have had a TIA, diagnostic tests will be done to determine the specific cause. In some cases you may be treated with drugs that can help prevent blood clots from forming, or your doctor may recommend surgery to open up a very narrowed carotid artery. If you have had a stroke, diagnostic tests will be performed and your doctor will decide upon the proper treatment. After a TIA, the goal is always to prevent a stroke from happening or returning.

One of the best ways to help prevent stroke is to correct some of the risk factors. The most important risk factor associated with stroke is hypertension, and the risk of having a stroke increases as the blood pressure increases. You can see how important it is to control high blood pressure as well as to try to change some of the other risk factors connected with a stroke.

EFFECT OF HYPERTENSION ON OTHER ORGANS

In addition to the cardiovascular system, high blood pressure can affect other organs, including the kidneys and the eyes.

As atherosclerosis affects the arteries in the kidneys, the blood flow to the kidneys is reduced. Over time, the kidneys can become damaged. Approximately 10% of all deaths due to hypertension result from kidney failure.

The blood vessels in the eyes can also become progressively narrowed. This can result in small *hemorrhages* (areas of bleeding) and swelling in the structures in the back portion of the eye responsible for vision. Your doctor can use the *ophthalmoscope* (a small instrument to view the back of the eye) to examine these blood vessels, and assess the effect the high blood pressure has had on these and other blood vessels throughout your body.

To sum up: untreated high blood pressure can affect your body and result in severe damage to your heart, your arteries, your brain, your kidneys, and your eyes. Understanding the consequences of untreated hypertension stresses the importance of keeping your blood pressure within a normal range. In the next chapter, we will review some of the other cardiovascular risk factors that often accompany high blood pressure, looking at some of the ways to modify these risks and help maintain the best state of health possible.

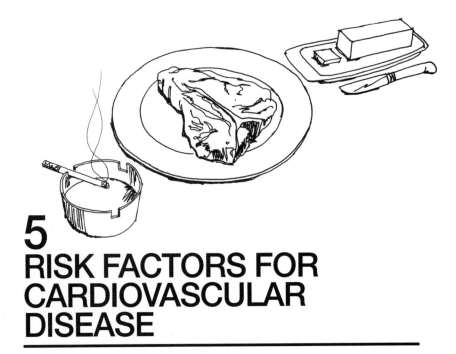

5
RISK FACTORS FOR CARDIOVASCULAR DISEASE

One of the more serious consequences of untreated hypertension is cardiovascular disease—diseases of the heart and blood vessels, including the arteries supplying the brain. Heart attacks and strokes are the most common of these diseases. High blood pressure is known to be the major risk factor associated with cardiovascular disease.

There are, however, other factors that can have a significant effect on the development of cardiovascular disease. In Chapter 3 we reviewed some of the factors that are associated with hypertension. Some of these same risk factors can increase your chance of developing other cardiovascular diseases by accelerating the development of atherosclerosis. The presence of a risk factor indicates that someone is more likely to develop cardiovascular disease than someone who has no risk factors. In addition, the presence of more than one risk factor greatly increases the chances of developing these diseases.

Some of these factors are permanent and can't be changed, while others can be. In this chapter we will review these risk factors and focus on ways in which you can work on those that can be modified, to help reduce the chance of developing cardiovascular diseases.

RISK FACTORS THAT CAN'T BE CHANGED

There are some factors we have no control over. These include our age, sex, and race. Many studies of heart disease and stroke have shown that increasing age is a risk factor for developing cardiovascular disease. In addition, there are also sex differences in the rates of these diseases. As a matter of fact, for people between the ages of 35 and 55, there is a five-fold higher death rate from cardiovascular diseases in men than in women. As described previously, there are also racial differences in the development of hypertension, with rates in blacks being twice as high as those in whites.

These are all factors which cannot be changed. Fortunately, there are other important factors which can be modified.

RISK FACTORS THAT MAY BE MODIFIED

Important risk factors include cigarette smoking, high cholesterol, and elevated blood fats (*lipids*), being overweight (*obesity*), elevated blood sugar (*diabetes mellitus*), stress, and physical inactivity. It is important to emphasize that you have a very important role in controlling or eliminating these risk factors.

CIGARETTE SMOKING

Many people are aware that cigarette smoking can cause damage to the lungs, including lung cancer, but are not aware of the major effect it has on the cardiovascular system. Cigarette smoking affects the heart, the blood vessels, and the blood components.

Smoking is known to speed up the process of atherosclerosis (thickening of the walls and narrowing of the arteries) throughout the body.

Cigarettes produce carbon monoxide (a poison), which is absorbed into the blood and body tissues replacing oxygen. Carbon monoxide can decrease the supply of oxygen to the heart and other organs and has damaging effects.

Cigarette smoking can affect the components in the blood and potentially alter the blood-clotting mechanisms.

Studies have shown that cigarette smoking is strongly associated with heart disease, diseases of the blood vessels, and with strokes. As a matter of fact, men who smoke cigarettes have about three to five times the risk of developing heart disease as those who don't smoke. Cigarette smoking also interacts with other risk factors to promote atherosclerosis.

There is encouraging news, however, because cigarette smoking is a risk factor that can be eliminated. Once you stop smoking there is a sharp drop in the risks associated with smoking—as quickly as within one year from the time you stop. The risk of deaths from other causes also decreases. Regardless of your age, quitting can improve your overall health and your life expectancy. **It is never too late to quit!**

If you smoke, you should ask your doctor or the American Heart Association chapter in your area about the different programs available that can help you stop smoking.

CHOLESTEROL AND OTHER FATS

You have probably heard the terms *cholesterol* and *unsaturated fats* many times over the last few years and have been told that low cholesterol is "good" and high cholesterol is "bad." What is cholesterol? What kind of fats are good and what kinds are bad? Can you control your cholesterol and fat levels by changing your diet?

Cholesterol and blood fats are known as blood *lipids*. An increase in cholesterol or fats is known as *hyperlipidemia*.

Cholesterol is a substance that is normally present in your blood. It is made mostly by the liver and carried in the blood by proteins to the different tissues in your body where it has many uses. The complex of cholesterol and protein is known as a *lipoprotein*. A certain amount of cholesterol is necessary for the body to carry out its normal functions.

Cholesterol is also present in many foods. These include egg yolks, red meat, and even certain kinds of shellfish. Although we need cholesterol, too much cholesterol in the blood and tissues is a risk factor for development of atherosclerosis of the blood vessels.

Scientists have discovered that there are really two kinds of cholesterol. The "good" kind of cholesterol is known as *HDL* (for high density lipoprotein), and the "bad" form is known as *LDL* (for low density lipoprotein). Increases in LDL appear to be a significant risk factor associated with cardiovascular diseases. HDL cholesterol is "good" cholesterol because it somehow protects against the development of plaques in the arteries.

In general, the higher the cholesterol level, the higher the risk of developing cardiovascular disease. As you can see, the amounts of each type of cholesterol is very important to consider. Your doctor will check the amounts and probably obtain a ratio of HDL cholesterol to total cholesterol. An HDL cholesterol of greater than 35 and a total cholesterol of less than 200 are thought to be reasonable levels.

Besides cholesterol, there are other fats (lipids) in the blood that can affect the process of atherosclerosis in the blood vessels. Our bodies need a certain amount of fat because fat provides us with energy. Like cholesterol, there are forms of fat that are good and forms that are bad. *Saturated fats* are unhealthy fats; *unsaturated fats* are helpful in that they can help lower the blood cholesterol. Saturated fats come from animal and dairy products such as meats, cream, cheese, and butter. Unsaturated fats are usually found in vegetable products and oils such as vegetable oil and olive oil. However, some non-animal oils such as coconut and palm oils are very high in saturated fats and are not healthy.

In the typical American diet, almost 40% of our food is fat. Fats also have twice as many calories as other foods such as protein and carbohydrates. Excess fat will affect your weight and your cholesterol level.

After your doctor evaluates your fat and cholesterol profile, he or she may recommend that you reduce the amount of cholesterol and saturated fats in your diet. Your doctor can recommend dietary changes, and you can also obtain information on dietary fats from your branch of the American Heart Association (see Appendix I). In general, foods that are low in cholesterol include fruits and vegetables, fish, breads and grains, low-fat yogurt, and cottage cheese. Your doctor may also suggest weight loss if you are overweight, because weight loss can decrease your cholesterol level. Daily exercise can also help to increase the "good" HDL cholesterol. If you do not respond to these measures, your doctor may use specific medications which act to lower blood lipid levels. By following the recommendations of your doctor and lowering your blood lipid levels, you will be helping to modify an important risk factor associated with cardiovascular disease.

EXCESS WEIGHT

Being overweight (obesity) is a risk factor associated with the development of cardiovascular diseases. Excess weight causes the heart to work harder to pump the blood throughout your body. Heart attack rates are increased in people who are 30% over their ideal body weight. Obesity can increase the development of atherosclerosis in blood vessels. In addition, obesity is closely associated with high blood pressure, high blood sugar, and high blood lipids. All these other risk factors, as you now know, compound the risk for developing cardiovascular diseases. Being overweight by 30 pounds decreases your life expectancy by 4 years.

Weight loss has many benefits. In general, it is associated with an overall feeling of better health for many people. It is often accompanied by a drop in blood pressure, blood fat and cholesterol levels are often lowered, and blood sugar often falls to lower levels. Losing weight will decrease the strain on your heart and enable you to be more active and maintain better cardiovascular fitness.

A balanced diet with an appropriate exercise program and support services is a well-rounded approach. You should discuss different weight loss programs with your doctor to ensure that they are safe for you and that they will meet your needs.

HIGH BLOOD SUGAR

Diabetes mellitus (diabetes) results in an increase in the amount of *glucose* (sugar) in the blood. Diabetes can be caused by too little *insulin,* the substance that is responsible for regulating the blood level of glucose. Some patients with diabetes can control their blood sugar by modifying their diets. Some need to take pills that help to regulate their blood sugar.

Others must inject insulin every day. The symptoms of diabetes can include excessive thirst, frequent urination, and weight loss. Your doctor can make the diagnosis by performing a series of blood tests which measure the metabolism of glucose in your blood.

Diabetes is a risk factor that is associated with cardiovascular disease. People with diabetes are two times more likely to have a heart attack than are people who don't have diabetes. Diabetes can increase the degree of atherosclerosis in the blood vessels, and can also affect other organs in your body, including the kidneys, the eyes, and the nerves. It is important to try to control your blood sugar if you have diabetes to help avoid the potential complications that may occur.

EXERCISE

According to some studies, people who get little or no exercise on the job or through their daily activities are more likely to have a heart attack. It is not really known how physical activity helps to prevent heart attacks and other cardiovascular diseases, but exercise can improve your body's fitness by:

- Improving your circulation and making your heart, lungs, and muscles work better together
- Making the heart pump blood more efficiently; the heart may pump more slowly, but more forcefully
- Improving your physical strength and muscle tone. You will tire less easily and may feel that you have extra energy
- Helping to maintain your ideal weight
- Often helping to reduce your blood pressure

Many people who exercise regularly say that they feel better mentally. They often find that they sleep better and, in general, feel more relaxed and able to handle stress and tension better. You should discuss your plans to exercise with your doctor so you can begin an appropriate fitness program.

STRESS

Everyone has some form of stress in their lives—relationships with others, tension on the job, children to raise, or bills to pay. Stress can come from outside influences or from internal causes such as depression or anxiety. Happy events, such as a wedding or buying a new home, as well as sad events, such as a loved one's death or loss of a job, can produce stress and worry. You can feel this stress both mentally and physically. During these periods of acute stress, your body may react in a number of different ways. Your heart may beat faster, and your blood pressure may rise in order to supply your heart and muscles with extra oxygen and nutrients. You may breathe more rapidly, taking in more oxygen.

Many people have the impression that stress is a risk factor associated with cardiovascular disease, but no one is really certain what role stress plays in cardiovascular disease. The way that people cope with stress may be important. Your general personality style over your lifetime may be a more important risk factor. The cigarette smoking and poor dietary habits that often accompany a stressful lifestyle may also play an important role.

In summary, high blood pressure is thought to be the most important risk factor associated with cardiovascular diseases. But when factors such as cigarette smoking and high cholesterol are linked with hypertension, the risk can be very great.

The good news is that many of these risk factors can be controlled. For example, knowing the substantial health risks often helps people to stop smoking. By doing so, your risks for developing various diseases decrease. You can also modify your cholesterol, your weight, and your level of physical activity. By doing so, you are working toward a longer and healthier life.

An encouraging fact is that the death rate from various cardiovascular diseases has been steadily declining over the last twenty to thirty years. The number of strokes has decreased dramatically. Most studies suggest that this decline is due to Americans controlling some of their risk factors. Most importantly, advances in the treatment of hypertension over the last twenty to thirty years are probably the most influential factor accounting for this decline.

In chapters to come, we will discuss the different means of controlling your blood pressure and stress the important role you will play in helping to maintain the best health possible.

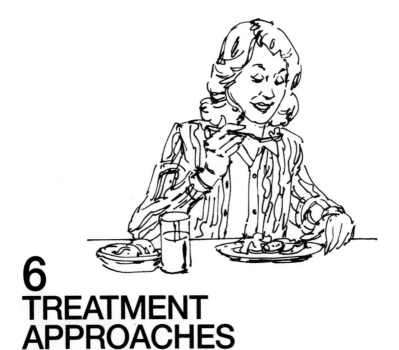

6
TREATMENT
APPROACHES

Physicians have learned a great deal about the treatment of hypertension in recent years. We have seen a great decline in cardiovascular diseases, including strokes, over the past twenty years, largely due to treating high blood pressure and controlling other risk factors. Today we really have no doubt that hypertension has many damaging effects on different organs of the body. We know that by controlling high blood pressure we can help reduce these complications.

Years ago, many people with "slightly high" blood pressure were not treated because doctors were not aware of the harmful effects over time of even mildly to moderately elevated blood pressure. These patients were monitored, but treatment was seldom prescribed. According to studies, however, people with even mild hypertension benefit from high blood pressure treatment. Studies indicate that they are less likely to have a stroke than those who are not treated. There may also be a reduction in other cardiovascular diseases. In addition, we know now that treating elevated systolic blood pressure (the top number in your blood pressure measurement) is just as important as treating elevated diastolic blood pressure (the bottom number in your blood pressure recording).

The knowledge that has led to many different forms of treatment of high blood pressure is relatively new. Years ago, very few medications were available. Often they were not fully effective in lowering blood pressure, and they frequently had many side effects. More than one medication was often required, and the dosing schedules were complicated. For these reasons, many people had a hard time remembering to take their medications or did not want to continue their treatments because of the bad side effects.

We are really much more fortunate today. We have come a long way in developing treatments for high blood pressure. The drugs that have been developed in recent years are more successful in lowering blood pressure than those of the past. They are also associated with fewer side effects and their schedules are much easier to follow. Today there are many different drugs that are available. Your doctor can choose the appropriate drug for you. In addition, there is much more known about the effects of other risk factors such as cigarette smoking and high cholesterol. There are now medications available to treat those cases of increased blood fats that are not responsive to diet alone.

In general, more cases of high blood pressure are being detected and treated than ever before.

METHODS OF TREATING HIGH BLOOD PRESSURE

Medical therapy using different drugs has been the main form of treatment of high blood pressure. Most patients will need only one or two different drugs to control their blood pressure adequately. In some cases, patients may need to be treated with multiple medications to keep their pressure in a reasonable range. Some people may have their blood pressure lowered effectively by other means, including weight loss, cutting down on salt, exercising, and relaxation techniques. Most often, a combination of medical and non-medical treatment is very effective. We will be describing these various forms of treatment in the chapters to come.

We previously reviewed the two different forms of hypertension: primary (essential) hypertension, and secondary hypertension in which there is often an underlying cause. We will be focusing primarily on the treatment of essential hypertension, which is the form that is found in approximately 90% of people who have high blood pressure.

As we stressed previously, there is no "cure" for this form of high blood pressure. Our goal, therefore, will be to control your blood pressure so that it remains in an acceptable range.

When many people first learn that they have high blood pressure, they become concerned that in order to treat it, they will have to rearrange their entire lives. This false belief unfortunately results in some patients stopping their therapy. The truth is that very few people with hypertension have to make substantial changes that interfere with their lives. Most of the changes that are recommended are not very difficult to accept, and will eventually blend right into your life as time goes on. The important thing to remember is that even if these changes do take some time getting used to, the benefits to your health far outweigh any small changes in lifestyle.

The particular program designed to treat your high blood pressure will depend on how high your blood pressure is, what other medical problems you may have, your age, your sex, and the presence of other cardiovascular diseases. The program will be individualized; that is, it will be tailored specifically to your needs. Your doctor will discuss these issues with you when you begin treatment.

You are beginning a long-term project whose goal is to control your blood pressure throughout your lifetime. You will be working closely with your doctor and with other health professionals. The aim of the treatment program will be for you to feel comfortable and confident about your role in managing your blood pressure. It may take some time and some changes to arrive upon the best program for you. The results are always worth it.

In the next chapter, we will review some of the non-drug therapies that may be useful in lowering your blood pressure. In the following chapter, we will focus on the different drug treatments that are currently available to treat hypertension.

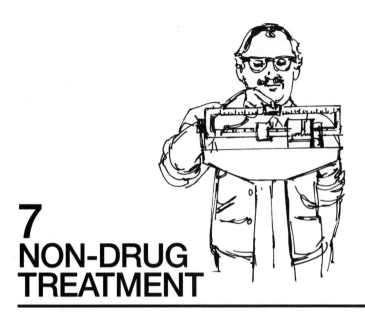

7
NON-DRUG
TREATMENT

Many different forms of therapy can help lower high blood pressure. In previous chapters we discussed some of the different cardiovascular risk factors that, when modified, may also help to lower blood pressure. These include weight reduction, exercise, cutting down on salt intake, and learning to better manage stress. If your blood pressure is only slightly high, these measures alone may be enough to bring your blood pressure down, although many patients will also need to take medication. In this chapter we will review the different forms of non-drug therapy that may be helpful in lowering your blood pressure.

WEIGHT LOSS

Although being overweight does not always result in high blood pressure, there is a strong relationship between the two. Overweight people are approximately three times more likely to have high blood pressure than persons of normal weight. Excess weight also places a greater burden on your heart. In addition, being overweight may make it harder to control your blood sugar if you have diabetes.

If you are overweight, your doctor will urge you to lose those extra pounds. If your weight is within normal limits, it is important for you to keep your weight there. Several studies have indicated that some people who are overweight will show a significant reduction in their blood pressure simply by losing weight.

For some people this may be the only treatment necessary, or it may be only the first step. If your blood pressure is only mildly elevated, your doctor may suggest a weight reduction program and then monitor your blood pressure to assess whether it is adequately controlled. If you require drug treatment, weight loss may mean fewer drugs or lower dosages.

The key will be to maintain your weight at a lower level. If you gain the weight back, the effects of weight loss are gone and your blood pressure is likely to increase again.

CONTROLLING YOUR DIET

Controlling your diet can be a positive move toward better health for many reasons. Changing your dietary intake can help you to lose unwanted extra pounds, and may help lower your cholesterol and blood lipids. If you also cut down on salt intake, this may help to lower your blood pressure. By changing your diet, you may help slow the process of atherosclerosis of the circulatory system.

After the age of 25, even if they eat the same kinds and amounts of food as before, people usually begin to gain weight. In general, the body needs 10 fewer calories a day for each year older than age 25. One hundred extra calories a day (about 10 potato chips) can add up to about 10 extra pounds a year! You can see how easy it is to put on weight if we don't modify our eating habits as we get older.

It is often helpful to think of weight in terms of supply and demand. If you supply your body with more food (calories) than the body needs without burning those calories off by exercise, you will gain weight. Your body's oversupply of calories will be deposited as fat. When you diet, the goal is to burn up the stored fat. To do this, you will need to cut down on calories in your daily meals and exercise.

Exercise increases the demand for, and helps to use up, the stored fat. Everyone's metabolism (the use of energy to keep the body running) is different. Some people can eat more and exercise less and still maintain a reasonable weight, while many people find that they will gain weight when they increase their caloric intake by even a small amount.

HELP IN DIETING

Losing weight can be very difficult. It can be even harder to keep the weight off once you have lost it. There is no sure way to lose weight, and individuals respond differently to various methods of weight loss. If you are overweight, it is most likely due to poor eating habits. Some of these habits are lifelong and can't be changed overnight. Different weight loss programs can help you to develop new and healthier eating habits, so you consume less food and establish a program of exercise that is suitable for you.

Many people try to diet on their own. If they become frustrated, they may give up. If you are seriously overweight, you should consider getting help from an organized dieting program where doctors, nurses, and dietitians can structure your eating habits and provide you with support. They can help to ensure that the foods you eat are still pleasurable. They can help you establish realistic goals regarding how much weight you should lose and how fast. You should avoid fad diets and crash diets; they can be dangerous to your health and seldom promote permanent weight loss.

In addition to professional assistance, many excellent self-help groups and publications are available. (See Appendix I.) You and your family can try new dishes that are lower in fats and unhealthy calories. Many books and magazines are available with recipes for delicious, healthy cooking. Your diet doesn't have to be dull.

CUTTING DOWN ON SALT

Salt (sodium chloride) is one of several important minerals required by the body. Salt occurs naturally or is added to many of the foods we eat. You probably know it best in the form of table salt, which is 40% sodium and 60% chloride. Our diet is really very heavy on salt. Most of us consume about 10 grams (or 2 teaspoons) of salt a day. Many people add a great deal of extra salt to all of their foods as a matter of habit, often before tasting their food. We really only need the small amount of sodium chloride that occurs naturally in the foods that we eat.

The relationship between high blood pressure and salt intake is not completely understood. We do know that excess sodium chloride causes the body to retain excess fluid. When this excess fluid is not eliminated by the body, it adds to the volume of blood in the circulation. This excess volume can increase the blood pressure. When the amount of fluid circulating through our system is reduced (which can occur with a lower salt concentration), blood pressure is often reduced. Although too much salt does not result in an increase in blood pressure in everyone, studies have shown that by decreasing the intake of sodium, blood pressure can be lowered in some cases. Today there are effective medications (called *diuretics*) that help to remove extra sodium and extra fluid from our circulation. They are often very effective in helping to reduce blood pressure, and they have made very strict sodium restriction unnecessary.

SOME RESTRICTION IS OFTEN RECOMMENDED

Treatment for hypertension often includes at least some restriction of salt. Most experts agree that severe salt restriction is usually not necessary. This type of diet is quite impractical and, when used alone, is usually not effective in lowering blood pressure to the desired range. It is more common to aim for a moderate restriction of salt in the diet—to about 1 teaspoon per day. This is the amount of salt that occurs naturally in foods, combined with the hidden salt that occurs in processed foods. Reducing salt intake can lower your blood pressure as much as 10 mm Hg in some cases. Sometimes this may be all that is necessary, or it may help reduce the number of medications used or lower the dosages. Your doctor can make recommendations regarding the role of salt restriction in the treatment of your high blood pressure.

A reduced salt diet doesn't have to be bland and tasteless. Many people even claim that the more natural taste of food is better. In some cases, you may have to give up some of the foods that you like that are really very high in salt content, but you will likely find other delicious foods that are lower in salt content that you can still enjoy.

SIMPLE GUIDELINES

If your doctor recommends sodium restriction as part of the treatment for your high blood pressure, there are a few simple guidelines that might help you to modify your eating habits and lifestyle. Reducing your salt intake to a teaspoon or less per day can be accomplished by following these steps:

- Buy fresh meats, poultry, fruits, and vegetables.
- Try to add little or no salt when you prepare foods. You can try other herbs and spices (garlic, basil, onion) or lemon juice for added flavor.
- Add little or no salt to food at your table.
- Avoid canned or processed foods such as canned vegetables and TV dinners.
- Avoid salty foods such as bacon, sausages, processed cheeses, ketchup, mustard, salad dressings, and luncheon meats.
- Avoid foods with other substances that are high in sodium, for example MSG (monosodium glutamate), which is used most frequently in oriental foods and in taste-enhancer products.
- Read the labels of the foods that you buy, paying attention to the sodium content.

By educating yourself about the salt content of different foods, you will be able to make informed decisions about which foods are healthy to eat and which have too much salt. The charts in Appendix II compare typical daily diets—one that is high in sodium and one that is low. In addition, there are some selected foods listed along with their salt content. They are not meant to be complete, but are included to show you the range of sodium content so you will know which foods are probably not healthy for you to eat on a regular basis.

Besides cutting down on salt, you may also be changing your dietary habits to include less cholesterol and saturated fats. If you feel you need some help in planning your diet, a dietitian can help you compile lists of healthy foods, and foods you should stay away from. This will help to ensure that your diet is nutritionally balanced as well as tasty.

In recent years, salt substitutes have become available on the market. They usually contain minerals other than sodium, such as potassium, in the form of potassium chloride. These can add the "salty" taste that many people like, and are sprinkled on your food as you would use salt. Potassium is an important mineral that you need in your diet, so these salt substitutes often are helpful in providing needed dietary potassium. You should always check with your doctor before you begin using them, however, since there are some medications used to treat high blood pressure that may also increase your potassium.

EXERCISE

Exercise is an important part of any program aimed at keeping you in good health. For many years, it has been recognized that some of the benefits of exercise include lowering blood pressure and improving the health of the circulatory system. In addition, exercise has other benefits which include reducing levels of fats and LDL ("bad") cholesterol, and increasing HDL ("good") cholesterol. Exercise helps with weight loss, can help you maintain your new weight, and help with depression and mood. In general, your physical strength is improved and you can do more and tire less easily. Many people will simply feel better and more relaxed after exercise.

The best exercise for your cardiovascular system is known as *aerobic* exercise. This type of exercise increases your heart rate and uses up energy. Aerobic exercises include walking, jogging, swimming, and bicycling. Many studies have shown that people with hypertension have a reduction in blood pressure when they are on a regular aerobic exercise program.

Before beginning any exercise program, you should discuss the program in detail with your doctor. He or she may pursue some simple tests of your heart's function to ensure that it is safe for you to begin. You should always start exercising very slowly and build up to the desired heart rate and degree of difficulty. Once your doctor gives you the OK, you are ready to choose the type of exercise program you want to do. You may decide to join a health club or gym, or you may choose to exercise on your own. Today there are many exercise machines that are available for home use, including exercise cycles and stair climbers. Whatever you choose to do, by exercising regularly you are helping to keep yourself in the best health possible.

RELIEVING STRESS

The relationship between high blood pressure and life stress is not really fully understood. Although there is no clear proof, there is the general impression that people with significantly stressful lifestyles are at a higher risk for developing cardiovascular disease. Some researchers feel it may not be the stress itself, but the mechanisms of coping with this stress that may be the important factor. In any case, learning to deal with stress may help to control your blood pressure better and will likely help you feel better in general. There are different techniques in use to help with relaxation which may have some effect on blood pressure. These include meditation, yoga, and biofeedback. As we previously noted, daily exercise can also serve as a means of stress reduction for many people. Although these methods are usually not effective in themselves for lowering blood pressure, they may help you as part of a well-balanced health and fitness program.

In this chapter, we reviewed several factors that may be modified to help control your blood pressure. Although they can be very beneficial and help to promote a general sense of well being, on their own they seldom control blood pressure adequately in most individuals. We discussed the benefits of a healthy diet, reducing the amount of cholesterol intake, and trying to avoid saturated fats. A very restricted intake of sodium is probably not necessary in most cases; however, cutting down on salt and being aware of the salt content of the foods you eat can be helpful in controlling your blood pressure. Exercise may help reduce your blood pressure, can help you maintain a healthy weight, and can help promote a general state of well-being. You should always discuss any change in your level of activity or any planned dietary changes with your doctor to ensure that they are safe for you.

In the next chapter, we will review the different medications presently used to control blood pressure.

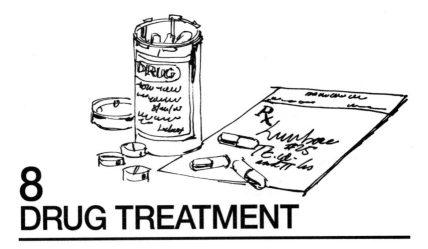

8
DRUG TREATMENT

There are many different medications available today that are used to treat hypertension. They often work by making adjustments in the mechanisms that regulate blood pressure. Each group of medications works on a different component of the blood pressure regulation system. Some tend to work better in certain individuals. The amounts needed to control blood pressure vary in different people. Because the drugs work on different blood pressure regulation systems, combining two or more different medications in patients with hard-to-control blood pressure is often very successful.

As you first begin treatment with a particular medication, your doctor will be watching your blood pressure very closely. During these early stages of treatment, your dosages may be changed often. You may be switched from one medication to another, or be placed on more than one medication. During this period, you will be working very closely with your doctor, whose goal will be to get your blood pressure under the best possible control while minimizing any potential side effects from the medication you are taking.

A SERIOUS PROBLEM

Unfortunately, many people begin their treatment for high blood pressure and then simply stop taking their medication. Studies find that 20 to perhaps 50 percent of patients may stop taking their blood pressure medication on their own sometime during their treatment. Let's review why some people are tempted to stop their treatment:

• Most people with high blood pressure don't feel sick. Many people associate taking medication with a particular symptom or illness (such as headache, ulcer or chest pain). Unfortunately, although most people will not feel the effects of their high blood pressure in the short term, there are many severe complications that develop when hypertension is not treated.

- Some people don't like to take drugs in general and subconsciously "forget" to take their medication.

- Some people think that taking medication for a short time will lower their blood pressure permanently and "cure" their hypertension.

- Drugs have side effects, including the drugs for high blood pressure. Often, people stop taking their medication because of unpleasant side effects. Some people don't know that if a side effect is troublesome, their doctor can often try a different medication or lower the dose.

- Some people are on many medications for many different illnesses. They may blame their blood pressure medications for making them feel sick.

- Some people feel their medication schedule is too complicated. In some cases, their doctors may not have explained in detail how to schedule multiple medications appropriately.

- Some people feel their medications are too expensive.

- Some people are afraid they will become addicted to drugs and do not want to take them. Drugs used to treat high blood pressure have not been found to be addicting.

We have stressed the importance of treating hypertension many times in this book, and by now you are aware of the many potential medical complications that can arise if high blood pressure is not lowered. If medications are part of your regimen to control your blood pressure, it is very important that you follow your doctor's orders and take your medications every day. If you are tempted for any reason to stop taking them, always talk it over with your doctor.

USING PRESCRIPTION MEDICATIONS

You may never before have taken prescription medications every day, on a permanent basis, and you probably have many questions about these drugs. Prescription drugs play an important role in modern medicine, but the subject of drugs and their proper use may seem very complicated. For example, many different drugs may serve the same purpose, while one particular drug may be used to treat many different kinds of illnesses. You may also hear one drug called by different names, which may be confusing to you.

We believe that you will find it easier to take your medications regularly if you understand why it is so important. It may help if you also understand a little bit about how medications work to lower your blood pressure. The mechanisms can be very complicated, since different medications work on different blood pressure regulation systems. It is also very important to be aware of side effects. Your doctor is familiar with the different blood pressure medications that are on the market. He or she will decide upon the appropriate medication for you based on your general medical profile, your medical history, and depending on what other medications you may be taking.

There are many reference sources your doctor may use that describe these medications in great detail, including possible side effects. Although your doctor will be making decisions regarding the appropriate drug for you, it is important for you to be as educated as possible about the drugs you will be taking. In this chapter, we will first introduce some general information about prescription drugs, then help you understand why it is so important to use these medications properly. We will then focus on how some of these medications work, and what some of the potential side effects are that you should be aware of.

IMPORTANT FACTS YOU SHOULD KNOW
ABOUT YOUR MEDICATIONS

There are several very important things that you should know about any drug that is prescribed for you. These include:
- The name of the drug or drugs
- Why you are taking the drug
- The dosing schedule—that is, the amount, the time to take it, and how often to take it
- Whether it has any serious side effects you should be aware of and what you should do if they occur
- Whether it will interact with any other drug you are presently taking
- Whether you must be careful about drinking alcohol or whether you need to avoid certain activities such as driving

FOLLOWING YOUR DRUG REGIMEN

Whenever you are prescribed a drug, your doctor will tell you the amount of the drug to take and how often to take it. Each drug works differently and should be taken in a specific manner. For example, some drugs may need to be taken with meals while other drugs are better absorbed on an empty stomach. Some drugs only need to be taken once a day, because their action is sustained over the entire day, while other drugs need to be taken more often. You should always take the precise amount of drug that your doctor prescribes. Some drugs won't work well unless the full amount is taken. Many drugs can be dangerous if more than the prescribed amount is taken. Some drugs must be stopped very gradually, over a period of time, and can be dangerous if stopped suddenly. It is important that you know what to do if you forget to take a dose; some medications can be taken later in the day when you remember.

All of these are issues that you should discuss with your doctor. You should never feel embarrassed about asking your doctor anything that is related to your illness or your medications. It is important for your doctor to know if your medication schedule is too complicated, or if you are having problems that may be related to one of the medications or to the combination of drugs that you are taking.

OTHER PRECAUTIONS

Before any drug is prescribed for you, your doctor will need to know other facts, such as whether you have any allergies or whether you have had any bad reaction to any drug in the past. Even though you might not think a particular fact is important, you should let your doctor know about any unusual reaction you may have had. You should let your doctor know if you are on a special diet. You should always let your doctor know if you are pregnant or if you may become pregnant, since this is an important consideration before choosing any drug. Some drugs, including birth control pills, vitamins, and cold remedies may interact with particular medications. You should always let your doctor know about all the medications you are taking. In addition, whenever you are given a new drug you should always ask your doctor if you will feel any differently or if it will interfere with your normal activities. For example, if the drug is likely to produce dizziness or sleepiness, you shouldn't drive or operate heavy machinery. Particular problems that may occur with medications for high blood pressure will be described later in this chapter.

SOME SAFETY TIPS FOR ALL DRUGS

There are a few important rules that should be applied to all medications to ensure safety:
- Keep all drugs out of the reach of children.
- If you are concerned that you have taken too many pills, or find pills missing from your bottles and suspect that you have taken an overdose, call your doctor or your local poison center immediately.
- Never give your medications to someone else. Likewise, never take anyone else's medications.
- Throw out drugs that are older than the expiration date on the label, and ask your doctor or pharmacist if you can throw out drugs that you no longer need.
- Always keep your labels on your medication bottles.
- Never mix medications in the same bottle.
- When you throw away medications, flush them down the toilet.

Don't throw them away into a wastebasket where someone else may find them.

MEDICATIONS FOR HIGH BLOOD PRESSURE

There are many medications available today to treat hypertension. As we previously noted, each class of drugs works on different components of the body's blood pressure regulation system. Appendix III lists many of the most commonly prescribed drugs. They are listed by their generic (chemical) names as well as by their brand or trade names. You may hear your doctor, nurse, or pharmacist refer to either or both of these names, so you should be familiar with both names of the drug that you are taking.

In the following paragraphs, we will review some of the mechanisms of action of some of the more common classes of drugs used to treat high blood pressure. If you are interested in a full list of all of the side effects and drug interactions, you should speak with your doctor.

SYMPATHOLYTICS: BETA AND ALPHA BLOCKERS

This class of drugs is used to treat high blood pressure because of their effect on heart function. Certain chemicals in your body act on so-called *alpha* and *beta receptors* in your heart and blood vessels. When the chemicals stimulate these receptors, blood pressure and heart rate increase. Beta and alpha *blockers* actually block the effects of chemicals in your body that raise your blood pressure. This results in a slower heart rate as well as a decrease in the force of contraction of the heart muscle. These changes are beneficial to the heart. In addition, blood pressure is decreased as blood is forced out of the heart and into the arteries with less force. If they are not effective alone, beta blockers are often combined with other kinds of blood pressure-reducing agents. This class of drugs is also used to treat other forms of heart disease, particularly after a heart attack, and can be helpful in treating migraine headaches.

In the past few years, many new beta blocker drugs have become available, each working by the same mechanism but differing in other ways. Some need to be taken a few times a day, while some of the newer agents need to be taken only once a day because their action lasts longer. In addition, some of the earlier drugs had side effects that some of the newer drugs no longer produce.

These drugs must be used with extreme caution in patients who have asthma, diabetes, or congestive heart failure. Your doctor will determine if these drugs are safe for you.

With the use of beta blockers, there can be side effects, such as dizziness, depression, nausea, and fatigue. Some patients also complain of sexual problems, such as the inability to have an erection. Many people tolerate these medications well, however. Remember, you should always discuss with your doctor any side effect or problem with your medication.

Beta blockers must never be stopped abruptly. If they are, the body can react by increasing the heart rate and blood pressure and causing other problems in your circulatory system. Always discuss the discontinuation of medications with your doctor.

CALCIUM CHANNEL BLOCKERS

Calcium channel blockers also act on specific chemical substances in the body. They block the action of chemicals that regulate calcium movement through the cells in the heart and the blood vessels. Through these changes, the workload on the heart is reduced and the blood pressure is lowered. Changes in the blood vessels that make it easier for the heart to pump blood through the body will also occur. These drugs are also commonly used to treat coronary artery disease (disease of the arteries supplying the heart). They are often used in combination with beta blockers or with some of the other blood pressure-reducing medications.

Many new forms of these drugs have been introduced in recent years. Some newer forms of calcium channel blockers have reduced side effects. Some are very easy to remember to take because they can be taken just once a day.

Many people tolerate these drugs very well. However, side effects can include dizziness, weakness, constipation, and nausea. Again, you should let your doctor know if you are having any problems tolerating your medications.

ACE INHIBITORS

These drugs prevent the action of a specific chemical substance in the blood called *Angiotensin Converting Enzyme* (or *ACE*) which normally serves to increase blood pressure. The important thing to know is that these drugs inhibit this enzyme, and they will lower your blood pressure through their effects on your kidneys and blood vessels. They also help to reduce the workload on the heart and are used to treat congestive heart failure. They are often used in combination with other blood pressure medications.

New forms of these drugs, which can be taken just once a day and are often very well tolerated, also have been introduced in recent years. Reactions can include skin rash, coughing, and kidney problems. Your doctor will likely monitor your blood during the initial stages of therapy to ensure that you are tolerating the drug well.

DIURETICS

These drugs act on the kidneys to help remove excess fluid and sodium from the body. They reduce the circulating blood volume and, in doing so, help reduce blood pressure. You may have heard them referred to as "water pills" or "fluid pills." Years ago, they were one of the only choices available to treat high blood pressure and were used routinely as the first-line drug when treatment began. Today, there are many more drugs available to lower blood pressure and many have fewer side effects. Diuretics are used, however, in combination with other blood pressure indications in some circumstances, and are commonly used to treat congestive heart failure. Side effects can include dizziness, skin rash, and dehydration.

VASODILATORS

These drugs act directly to relax the smooth muscle located within the walls of blood vessels, resulting in lower blood pressure as well as a reduction in the workload of the heart. These drugs are not used often as a first choice to treat high blood pressure but are used frequently in combination with other agents. They are also used to treat congestive heart failure. Some of the drugs in this class are used in the emergency treatment of extremely high blood pressure.

The above descriptions of some of the more commonly used blood pressure medications were not meant to include all drugs available today, but to describe to you the way some of the more common drugs act to help control your blood pressure. Your doctor can provide you with information about the specific medications that you are taking.

BLOOD PRESSURE MEDICATIONS AND SIDE EFFECTS

Medications used for hypertension are capable of producing side effects. Many of these are minor and may not even be noticeable. It is important that you are aware of the possible side effects of the medications you are taking. In addition, you should always know about potential interactions if you are taking two or more drugs. It is important that you keep in mind that many people develop only mild side effects, and many others have no problems tolerating their medications at all.

Some patients feel different when they first start their blood pressure medications. As the body gets used to a drug, side effects often disappear. If you develop side effects that persist or can't be tolerated, your doctor may first try changing the dosage. If you are still having problems with your medication, your doctor may try another. There are many different kinds of drugs available on the market today, and it is very likely that your doctor will find the medication that is just right for you.

One problem that is found with many drugs that are used to treat hypertension is known as *orthostatic hypotension*. (Hypotension means low blood pressure.) This condition results in a dizzy, lightheaded, or woozy feeling when you get up suddenly from the lying or sitting position. Normally, when you arise quickly, your body is able to adjust your blood pressure to the appropriate level. Some medications used to treat hypertension make it more difficult for your body to make the rapid adjustments necessary. Occasionally, you can even faint. Sometimes orthostatic hypotension disappears after a few days, but occasionally it becomes a persistent problem. You should let your doctor know if you experience this problem.

Other common side effects include tiredness, mood changes, depression, and sexual problems. These can include a lack of desire or impotence. A dry mouth, cough, or stuffy nose can also occur with some medications. If you experience any of these problems, you should always discuss them with your doctor. You should never feel embarrassed about any side effects or any other symptoms you might be experiencing. For most people there are solutions that can help you better tolerate these side effects.

FINDING THE RIGHT COMBINATION

Your doctor will begin treating your high blood pressure with a medication that he or she feels is best for you. The plan of therapy will be individualized for you, taking into account your blood pressure measurements, your other medical problems, and what other medications you may be taking. The initial goal will be to lower your blood pressure using the least number of drugs and the lowest dosages possible.

After your doctor starts you on a medication, he or she will monitor the effect on your blood pressure. If your blood pressure is under control and you are tolerating the medication, you will likely continue on it. If your blood pressure is still too high, your doctor will first try increasing the dose. If your pressure is still not under control, a second medication may be added. In some cases, your doctor may decide simply to switch to another medication. Your doctor will continue to adjust your medications until your blood pressure is under the best control possible.

TAKING OTHER MEDICATIONS

Some of the medications that you can buy over the counter (without a prescription) can interfere with your blood pressure control. These include nasal sprays, cold remedies, and diet pills. Some antacids are very high in sodium. Some medications will have warnings on the label indicating that you are not to take them if you have high blood pressure. However, since not all medications have this information prominently displayed, to be safe you should always check with your doctor or pharmacist before taking any other medications.

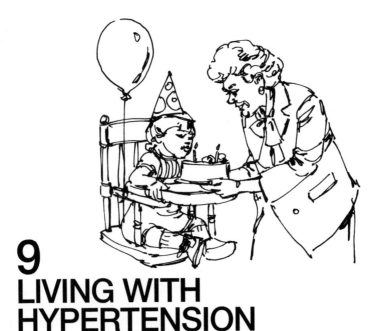

9
LIVING WITH HYPERTENSION

In this book, we have described many aspects of high blood pressure. In the early chapters, we reviewed the mechanisms that regulate normal blood pressure and how the body's systems can cause high blood pressure. Risk factors for high blood pressure and other cardiovascular diseases were discussed. We stressed the importance of treating high blood pressure in order to avoid the many potential medical complications that can result from untreated hypertension.

All of these facts may seem complicated in some ways. It all may be new to you, and you may feel overwhelmed by the large amount of information you think you need to know. In many ways, though, your job is simple. The most important things for you to remember are these:

- Accept the fact that you have high blood pressure and understand that it is often a lifelong condition.
- Realize the importance of controlling your high blood pressure and the benefits to your health of doing so.
- Take your medications daily as your doctor prescribes.
- Visit your doctor regularly to have your blood pressure monitored.
- Discuss any questions or issues with your doctor, and keep your doctor informed of any issues relating to aspects of your health.

You may be concerned that controlling your blood pressure will take up a great deal of time visiting doctors and taking medications. Actually, once your doctor finds the best treatment for your high blood pressure, you will likely be on a stable drug treatment program and may not have changes made very often. Your doctor will schedule follow-up visits to monitor the effects of treatment. During this time, you may start changing certain aspects of your lifestyle to modify some of the risk factors for high blood pressure and other cardiovascular diseases. This may include a new diet, beginning an exercise program, and stopping cigarette smoking.

Making these changes may be difficult at first, but in the long run, they will be of great benefit to your health. If you have difficulty on your own, ask for assistance. As we previously noted, formal exercise or diet programs are often very helpful. We think you will really feel better as you achieve these goals.

REMEMBERING TO TAKE YOUR PILLS

Many people find it hard to remember to take their medications at the appropriate times each day. Some people find it helpful to make a chart that lists the specific times that they need to take their medications. Other people leave notes around the house reminding them when to take their pills. For some people, involving family members can be very helpful. They can be an important part of your treatment program. There are also medication containers available that have separate compartments for each dose and day of the week. It is most important to make taking your medications part of your daily routine. Today, there are many new blood pressure medications available that need to be taken only once a day. Your doctor may recommend one of these longer-acting drugs for you.

If you are planning to go on vacation or are changing your daily routine, make sure that you have the needed supply of all of your medications. Before leaving home, you should determine the amount of medication that you need, and be sure to have your prescriptions refilled if needed. If you are traveling by airplane or boat, don't store your medication with your luggage. Always carry it with you to ensure that even if you are separated from your baggage, you will have your medication with you.

BLOOD PRESSURE MEASUREMENT AT HOME

Many patients ask whether they should be measuring their blood pressure at home. For many people who are taking medications and modifying other aspects of their lifestyle to control their hypertension, taking their blood pressure at home can reassure them that their treatment program is working and provide encouragement to continue. Blood pressure measurements taken at home may sometimes be a more accurate measure of a patient's blood pressure than measurements taken in a doctor's office. This is because patients are often anxious in a doctor's office or hospital, and this may result in higher blood pressure recordings.

Today, there are many easy-to-use devices available to measure blood pressure in your home. Some of them require very little skill and often record blood pressure in a digital readout. Your doctor can help you decide which model is best for you. If you do decide to buy a machine, be sure that you know how to use it accurately before you take it home. Your doctor or nurse can also help you learn how to take your own blood pressure.

Some doctors feel that home blood pressure monitoring is not necessary. You should discuss this with your doctor. If you do buy a monitor, it is very important that you remember never to change any of your medications because of measurements you obtain when you record your own blood pressure. Only your doctor should adjust your medications.

A SUCCESSFUL FUTURE

The important thing to remember is that you can learn to live with high blood pressure. By trying to learn as much as you can about high blood pressure and by taking an active interest in these issues, we feel that you will find living with hypertension much easier. With only a few exceptions, high blood pressure can be lowered and kept under control. The most important ingredient for successful control of hypertension, and for continued good health, is *you.* If you believe that your health is important, and believe in yourself, you will truly achieve success.

Loving your health is loving your life and your future.

APPENDIX I

INFORMATION SOURCES

1. An excellent booklet on losing weight, *Are You Really Serious About Losing Weight?* is available, directly through the publisher: PM Incorporated, P.O. Box 10172, Van Nuys, California 91410. This information is updated regularly to include the latest on weight loss in general and on special diets for people with heart disease, high blood pressure, and diabetes. The 64-page booklet contains realistic and encouraging advice plus many useful charts and tables.

2. Your local chapter of the American Heart Association can provide the following publications on dietary fats: *Cholesterol and Your Heart (Rev. 1992); Nutritional Labeling: Food Selection Hints for Fat Controlled Meals (Rev. 1992); Recipes for Fat Controlled Low Cholesterol Meals from the American Heart Association Cookbooks (Rev. 1992).*

3. *Good Cholesterol, Bad Cholesterol,* by E.M. Roth, M.D., F.A.C.C. and S.L. Streicher, R.N., Prima Publishing, California, 1990 ($9.95). This is a practical and user-friendly book which shows the reader how to adapt to a low-cholesterol lifestyle. Every aspect is covered from how to read labels, to eating out, to understanding the benefits and side effects of cholesterol-lowering drugs.

4. *Salt, Sodium and Blood Pressure,* a pamphlet available from the American Heart Association, provides guidelines for avoiding foods high in sodium, shows you how to find out the sodium content of various foods, and shows that reducing sodium in foods you eat may be easier than you think.

5. *Facts About Potassium,* a pamphlet available from the American Heart Association, lists the sodium content and calories in potassium-rich foods.

6. *Living Heart Diet,* by R. DeBakey, M.D., Simon & Schuster, Inc., 1984 ($13.00) is a clear, sensible, low-calorie, low-cholesterol diet plan developed by America's foremost heart surgeon. It contains more than 500 medically tested recipes for everything from appetizers to desserts along with a table for each recipe giving the precise levels of calories, fat, cholesterol, etc.

7. *About Your Heart and Exercise* is a booklet available from the American Heart Association which shows how to increase fitness, how to choose an exercise program, and how to start and continue with a program. It also includes an exercise log and calorie-use chart.

APPENDIX II

SAMPLE HIGH- AND LOW-SODIUM MENUS*

HIGH IN SODIUM   LOW IN SODIUM

Breakfast

1 cup cocoa, from		1 cup orange juice	5 mg
dry mix	232 mg	1 cup puffed wheat	
3/4 cup instant oatmeal		or rice cereal	1 gm
with maple and		1/2 cup milk	60 mg
brown sugar	277 mg	banana	2 mg
1 slice Canadian bacon	394 mg	cinnamon sweet roll,	
1 slice toast with butter	230 mg	frozen	110 mg

Lunch

1 fish sandwich		1 peanut butter sandwich	
(fast food)	882 mg	on white bread	309 mg
1 dill pickle	928 mg	apple	2 mg
10 potato chips	200 mg	1 cup yogurt with fruit	113 mg

Dinner

3 oz. ham	1114 mg	3 oz. pork chop	60 mg
1 cup mashed potatoes,		baked potato	5 mg
instant	485 mg	with sour cream	12 mg
with butter	116 mg	3 oz. frozen spinach	65 mg
1/2 cup canned spinach	455 mg	salad with 1 tbsp.	
salad with 1 tbsp.		French dressing,	
French dressing,		home recipe	92 mg
bottled	214 mg	1 slice frozen banana	
1/2 cup chocolate		cream pie	90 mg
pudding, instant	470 mg	(before adding salt)	946 mg
(before adding salt)	5997 mg		

---

* Sodium is measured in *milligrams*, abbreviated mg. One thousand milligrams equals 1 gram, or about one-fifth teaspoon.

(continues on next page)

(continued from previous page)

SODIUM CONTENT OF SELECTED FOODS

HIGHER IN SODIUM		LOWER IN SODIUM	
5 oz. chicken, canned	714 mg	7 oz. chicken, roasted	138 mg
Big Mac	1510 mg	hamburger, bun, lettuce and tomato, homemade	200 mg
2 oz. dried beef	2440 mg	3 oz. fresh beef	55 mg
3 oz. shrimp, canned	1955 mg	3 oz. shrimp, fresh	137 mg
2 frankfurters	1278 mg	3 oz. haddock	150 mg
meatloaf TV dinner	1304 mg	Swiss steak TV dinner	682 mg
turkey pot pie, frozen	1018 mg	turkey pot pie, homemade	620 mg
1 cup vegetable beef soup from dry mix	1000 mg	1 cup vegetable beef soup, low sodium	51 mg
1 cup canned tomato soup	932 mg	1 cup canned tomato soup, low sodium	29 mg
1 cup canned split pea soup	987 mg	1 cup dried split peas	5 mg
1 cup kidney beans, canned	844 mg	1 cup dried kidney beans	4 mg
1 cup beets, canned	479 mg	1 cup broccoli, frozen	35 mg
1/2 cup mushrooms, canned	484 mg	1 cup mushrooms, raw	7 mg
1 cup sauerkraut	1554 mg	1 cup cabbage, raw	8 mg
1 cup carrots, canned	386 mg	1 carrot, raw	34 mg
1 cup creamed corn, canned	671 mg	2 ears corn on the cob	2 mg
1 cup tomatoes, canned	390 mg	2 tomatoes, raw	28 mg

HIGHER IN SODIUM		LOWER IN SODIUM	
1 dill pickle	928 mg	1 cucumber	14 mg
1 cup vegetable juice cocktail	887 mg	1 cup apple cider	5 mg
4 green olives	323 mg	3 black olives	96 mg
1 tbsp. soy sauce	1029 mg	1 tbsp. catsup	156 mg
1 tbsp. butter, salted	116 mg	1 tbsp. butter, unsalted	2 mg
1 oz. American cheese	406 mg	1 oz. cheddar cheese	176 mg
4 oz. cottage cheese	457 mg	4 oz. cottage cheese, unsalted	14 mg
1 cup Rice Krispies	340 mg	1 cup puffed rice	1 mg
1 cup Wheaties	355 mg	1 biscuit Shredded Wheat	3 mg
1 biscuit from mix	272 mg	1 brown and serve roll	138 mg
1 cup stuffing mix, cooked	1131 mg	1 cup noodles, cooked	2 mg

POTASSIUM AND POTASSIUM SUPPLEMENTS

Some Foods That Are High In Potassium

bananas	potatoes	chicken
orange juice	flounder	soybeans
melons	broccoli	molasses
grapefruit juice	raisins	nectarines
prune juice	strawberries	spinach
avocados	squash	veal

(continues on next page)

(continued from previous page)

POTASSIUM SUPPLEMENTS

Brand Names: Slow-K, Kay-Ciel, K-Lor, Kaon, and several others.

Form: Liquid, tablet, or powder.

How to take: With or following foods. When taken on an empty stomach, potassium can have a mild laxative effect or cause an upset stomach.

Precautions: Let your doctor know immediately if you have stomach pain and indigestion or if you notice blackish stools or other signs of intestinal bleeding. If you have trouble swallowing the tablets, tell your doctor.

Note: Potassium supplements should not be used unless recommended by your doctor. They can be dangerous if you have certain kidney problems or are using potassium-retaining diuretics.

APPENDIX III

COMMON MEDICATIONS USED FOR HYPERTENSION

**Common or
generic names**

**Some commonly used
brand names**

DIURETICS

Thiazide diuretics

bendroflumethiazide	Naturetin
benzthiazide	Exna
chlorothiazide	Diuril
chlorthalidone	Hygroton
hydrochlorothiazide	Esidrix, HydroDIURIL, Oretic
hydroflumethiazide	Diucardin, Saluron
indapamide	Lozol
methyclothiazide	Aquatensen, Enduron
metolazone	Diulo, Zaroxolyn, Mykrox
polythiazide	Minizide
quinethazone	Hydromox
trichlormethiazide	Metahydrin, Naqua

Loop diuretics

bumetanide	Bumex
ethacrynic acid	Edecrin
furosemide	Lasix

Potassium-sparing diuretics

amiloride hydrochloride	Midamor
spironolactone	Aldactone
triamterene	Dyrenium

(continues on next page)

(continued from previous page)

VASODILATORS

hydralazine	Apresoline
diazoxide	Hyperstat IV
nitroglycerin	Tridil, Nitro-Bid IV
minoxidil	Loniten
sodium nitroprusside	Nipride, Nitropress

SYMPATHOLYTICS

Beta Blockers

acebutolol	Sectral
atenolol	Tenormin
betaxolol	Kerlone
carteolol	Cartrol
esmolol	Brevibloc
labetalol	Trandate, Normodyne
metoprolol	Lopressor, Toprol XL
nadolol	Corgard
penbutolol	Levatol
pindolol	Visken
propranolol	Inderal, Inderal LA
timolol	Blocadren

Alpha Blockers

prazosin	Minipress
terazosin	Hytrin
doxazosin	Cardura

Others

clonidine	Catapres
deserpidine	Harmonyl
guanabenz	Wytensin
guanadrel	Hylorel
guanethidine	Ismelin
guanfacine	Tenex
methyldopa	Aldomet
Rauwolfia serpentina	Raudixin
reserpine	Serpasil

COMBINATION MEDICINES

hydrochlorothiazide & spironolactone	Aldactazide
chlorothiazide & methyldopa	Aldoclor
hydrochlorothiazide & methyldopa	Aldoril
hydrochlorothiazide & hydralazine	Apresazide, Apresoline-Esidrex
hydrochlorothiazide & captopril	Capozide
chlorthalidone & clonidine	Combipres
bendroflumethiazide & nadolol	Corzide
chlorthalidone & reserpine	Demi-Regroton
chlorothiazide & reserpine	Diupres
methyclothiazide & deserpidine	Diutensen-R
hydrochlorothiazide & triamterene	Dyazide
methyclothiazide & reserpine	Enduronyl
hydrochlorothiazide & guanethidine	Esimil
benzthiazide & reserpine	Exna-R
quinethazone & reserpine	Hydromox-R
reserpine & hydrochlorothiazide	Hydropres
hydrochlorothiazide & propranolol	Inderide
hydrochlorothiazide & triamterene	Maxzide
polythiazide & prazosin	Minizide, Renese
hydrochlorothiazide & amiloride	Moduretic
hydrochlorothiazide & deserpidine	Oreticyl
hydrochlorothiazide & deserpidine	Oreticyl Forte
bendroflumethazide & Rauwolfia serpentina	Rauzide
chlorthalidone & reserpine	Regroton
hydroflumethiazide & reserpine	Salutensin
hydroflumethiazide & reserpine	Salutensin-Demi
hydrochlorothiazide & reserpine & hydralazine	Ser-Ap-Es
chlorthalidone & atenolol	Tenoretic
hydrochlorothiazide & timolol	Timolide

61

CALCIUM CHANNEL BLOCKERS

amlodipine besylate	Norvasc
nifedipine	Procardia
nifedipine GITS	Procardia XL
nifedipine corecoat	Adalat CC
diltiazem	Cardizem, Dilacor XR
verapamil hydrochloride	Calan, Isoptin, Verelan
nicardipine hydrochloride	Cardene
felodipine	Plendil
isradipine	DynaCirc

ACE INHIBITORS

captopril	Capoten
enalapril maleate	Vasotec
lisinopril	Prinivil, Zestril
fosinopril sodium	Monopril
benazepril hydrochloride	Lotensin
quinapril hydrochloride	Accupril
ramipril	Altace

Notes

Notes

Notes

Notes

Notes

Notes

Notes

Notes

Notes

Notes

Notes

Notes